No Head Fred Said, "Send Thanks"

To Fisher Grandkids

Stephanie Keegan

STEPHANIE KEEGAN

PAGE PUBLISHING, INC.
Conneaut Lake, PA

First originally published by Page Publishing 2019

ISBN 978-1-64350-756-9 (pbk)
ISBN 978-1-64350-757-6 (digital)

Printed in the United States of America

Acknowledgement

Thank you to my parents Chris and Jim Barton.

A special thank you to Laurie (VanWey) Duncan for all the help with the books. And thank you to all who have supported No Head Fred.

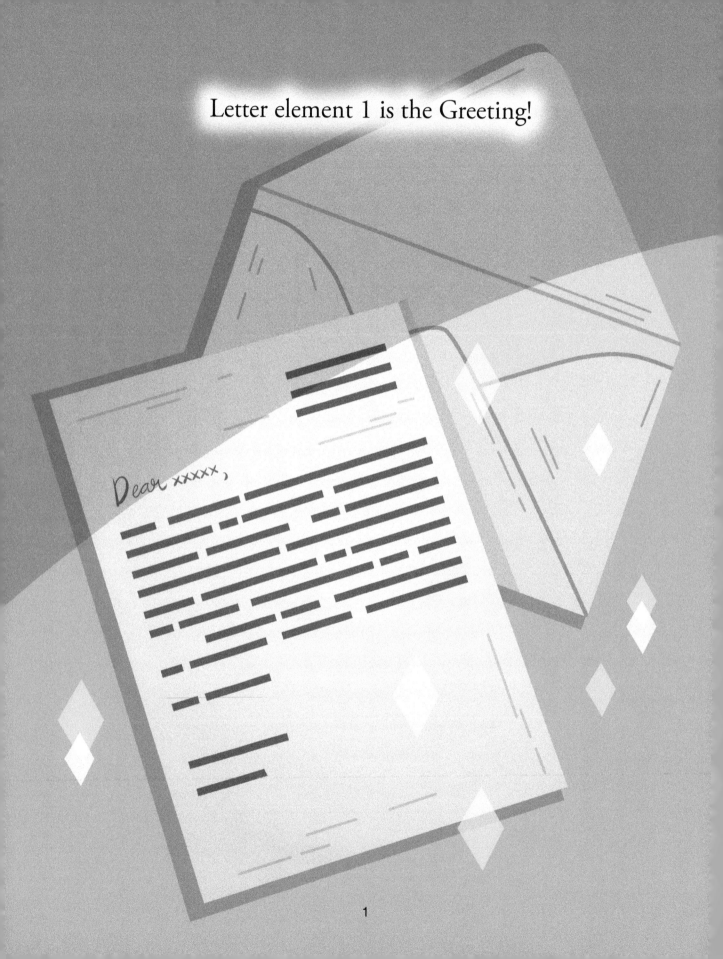

Letter element 1 is the Greeting!

Dear xxxxx,

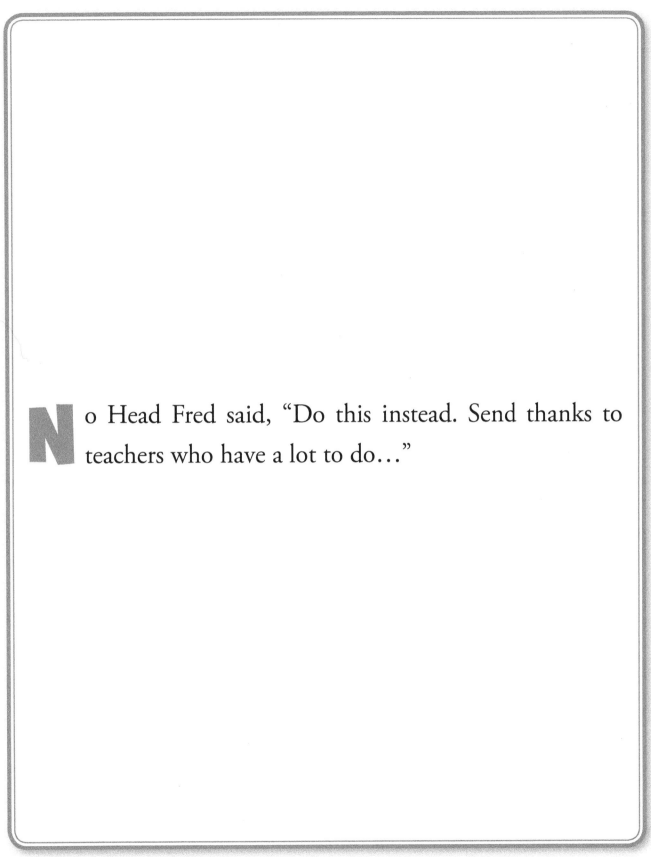

No Head Fred said, "Do this instead. Send thanks to teachers who have a lot to do…"

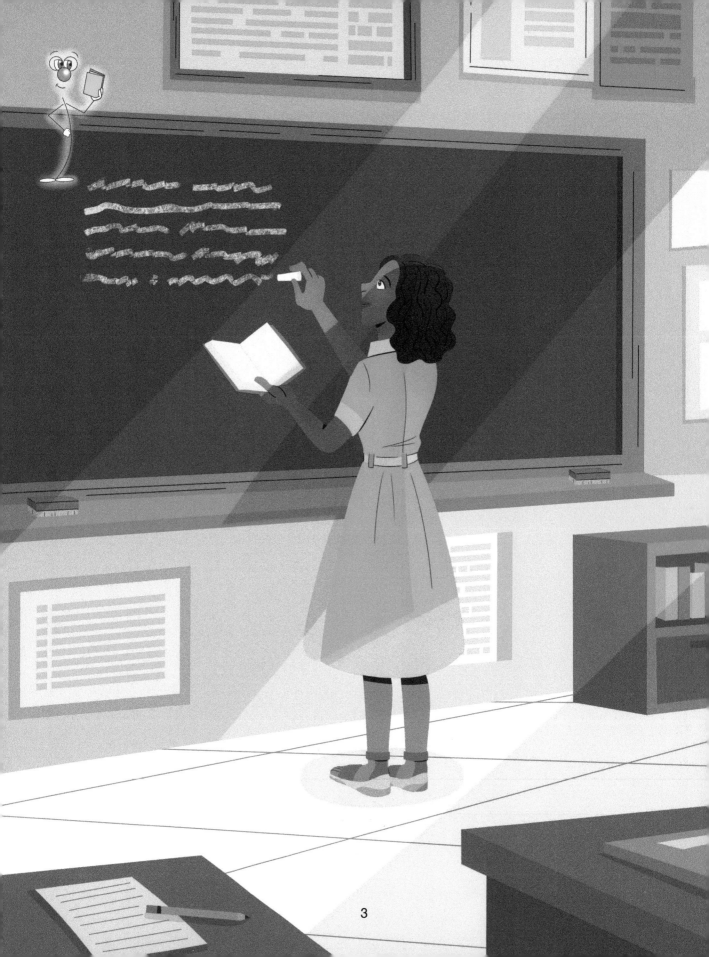

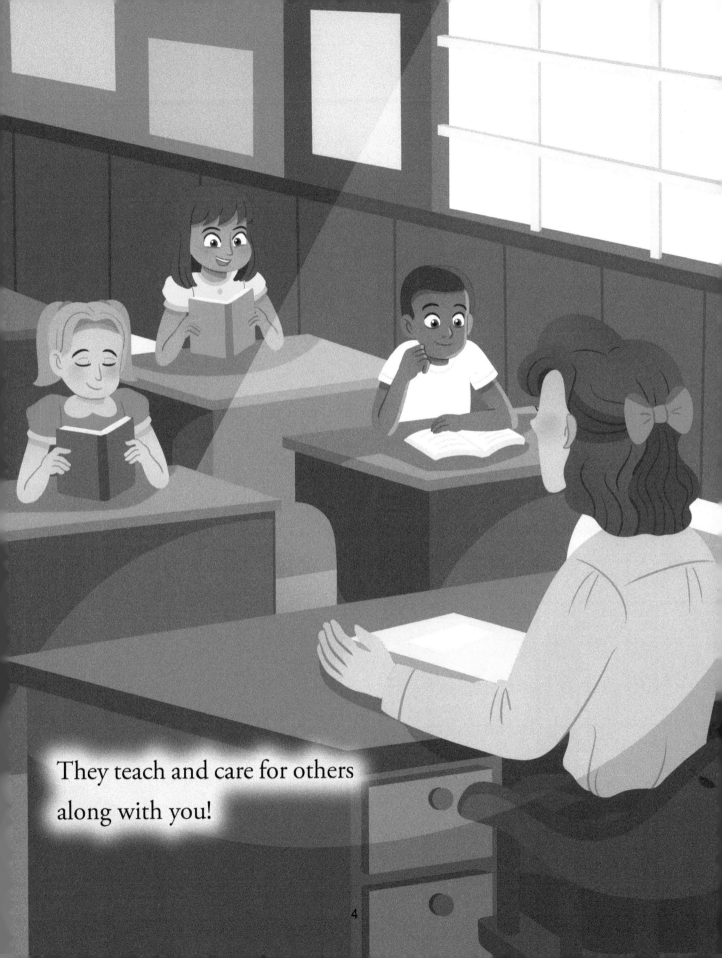

They teach and care for others along with you!

Letter element 2 is the Body!

Thank you for ×××××

No Head Fred said, "Do this instead. Send thanks to police who face danger every day…"

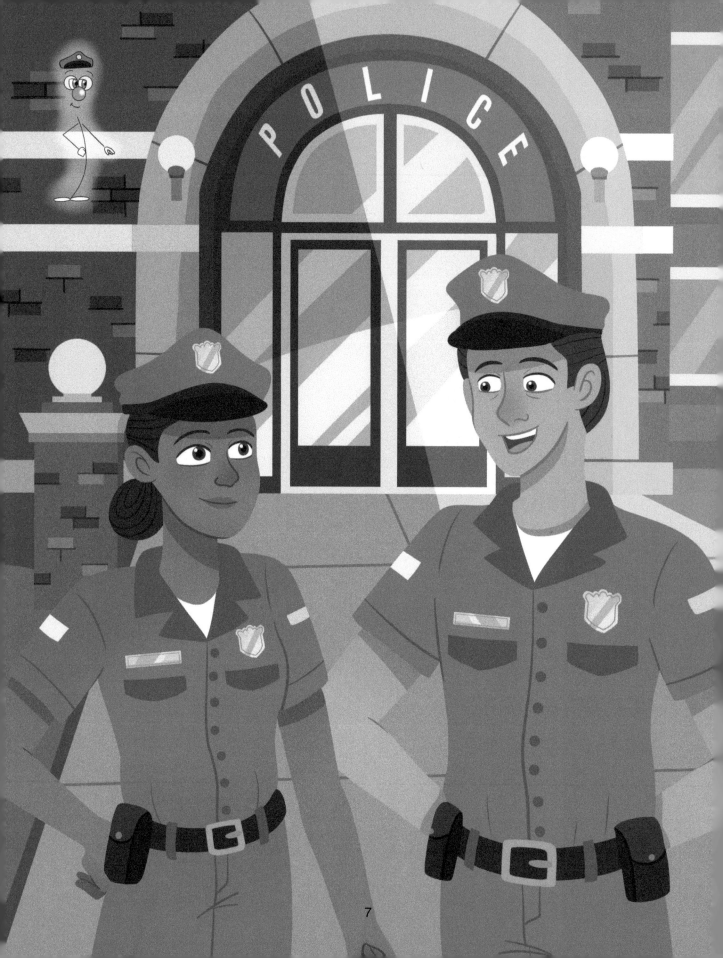

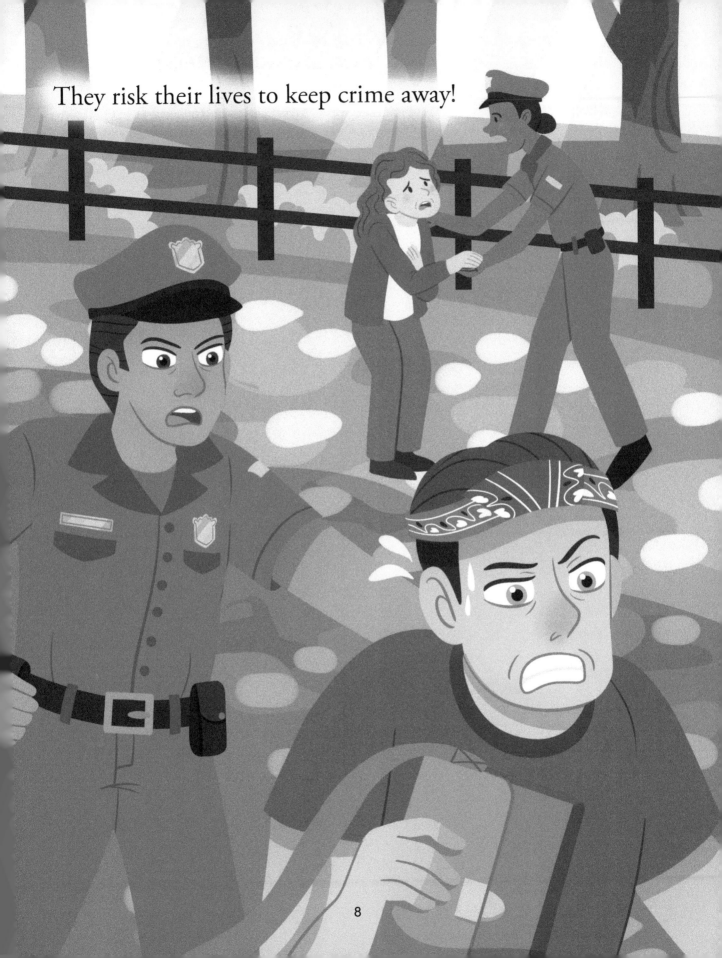

They risk their lives to keep crime away!

Letter elements 3 and 4 are the Closing and Signature!

Sincerely xxxxxx.

No Head Fred said, "Do this instead.

Send thanks to firefighters who are always on call…"

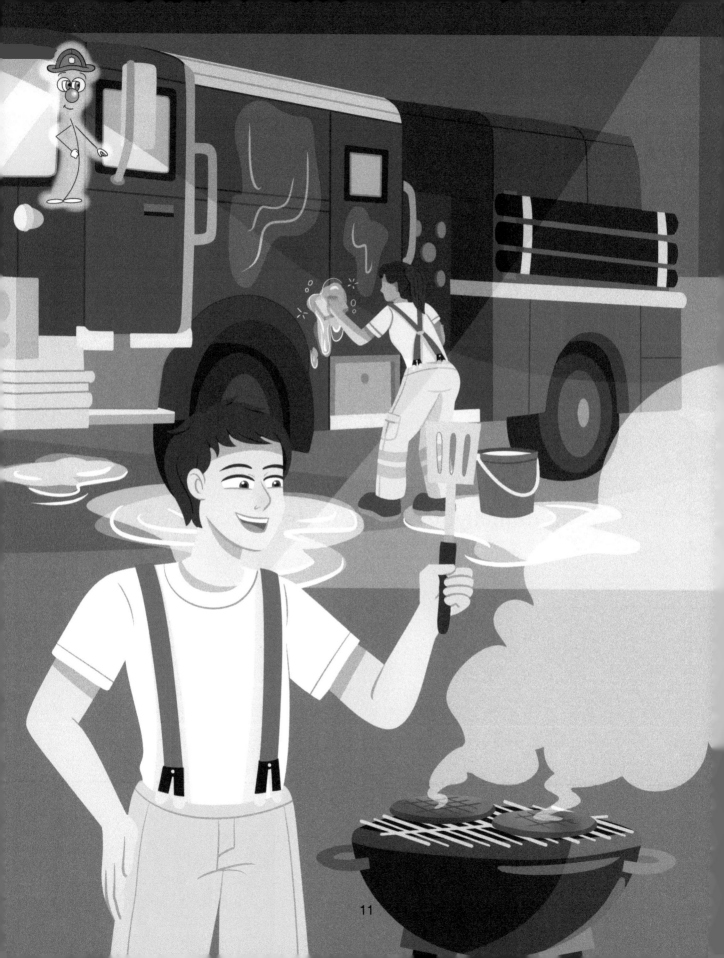

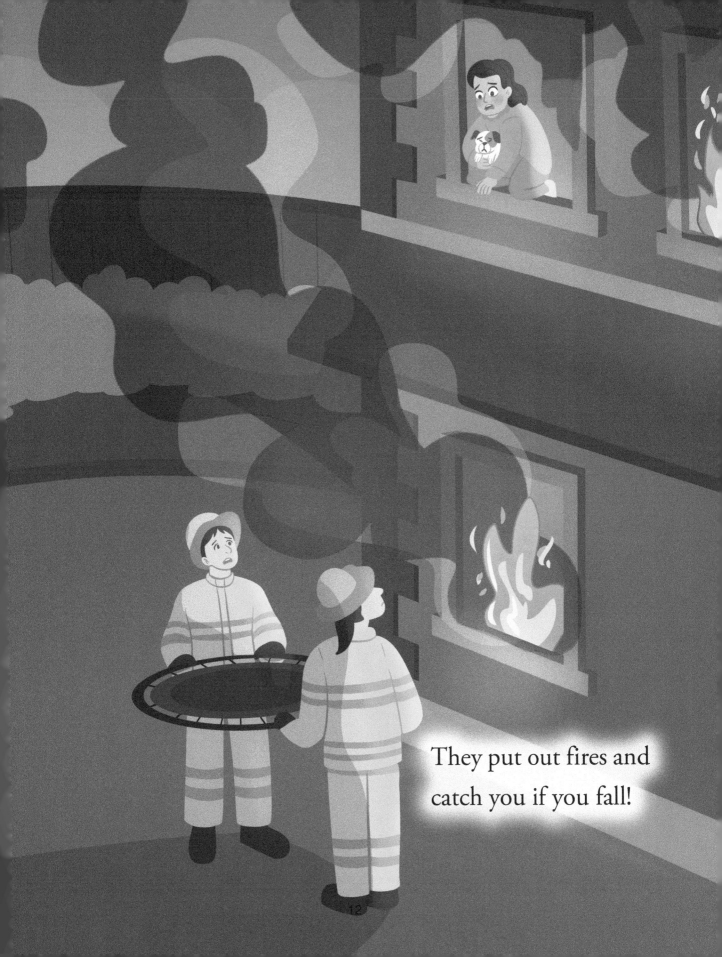

They put out fires and
catch you if you fall!

12

No Head Fred said, "Do this instead. Send thanks to the coast guard, army, navy, air force, and marines..."

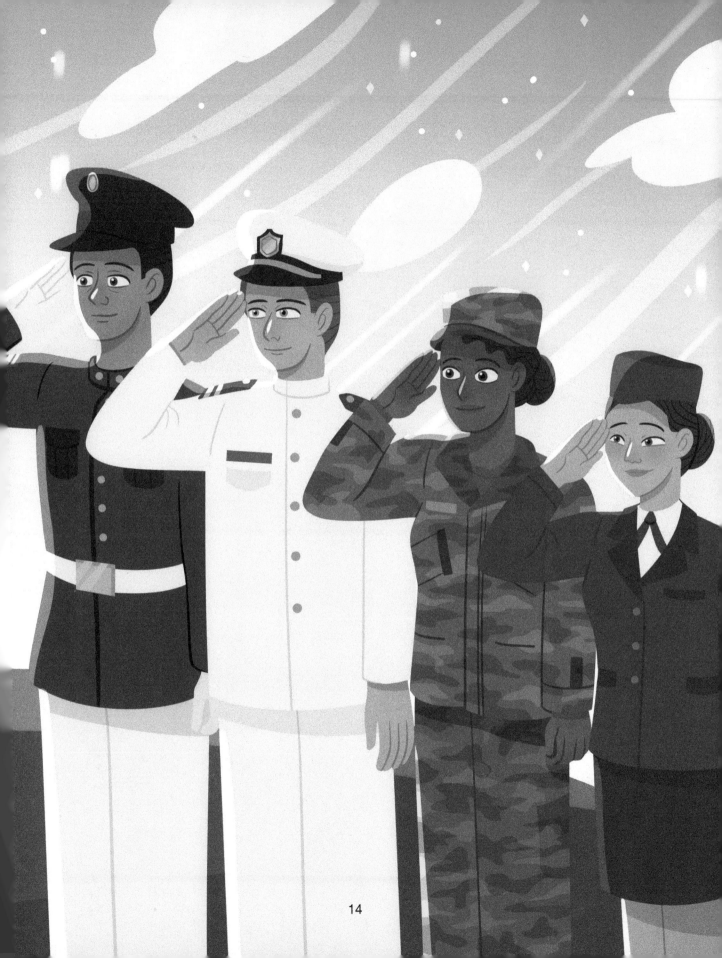

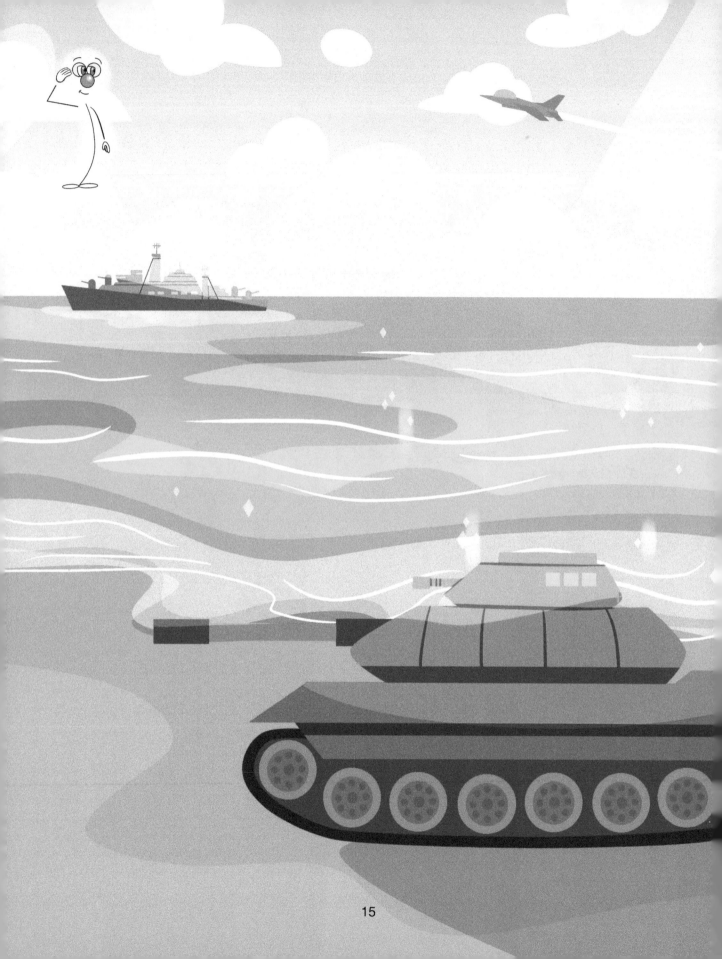

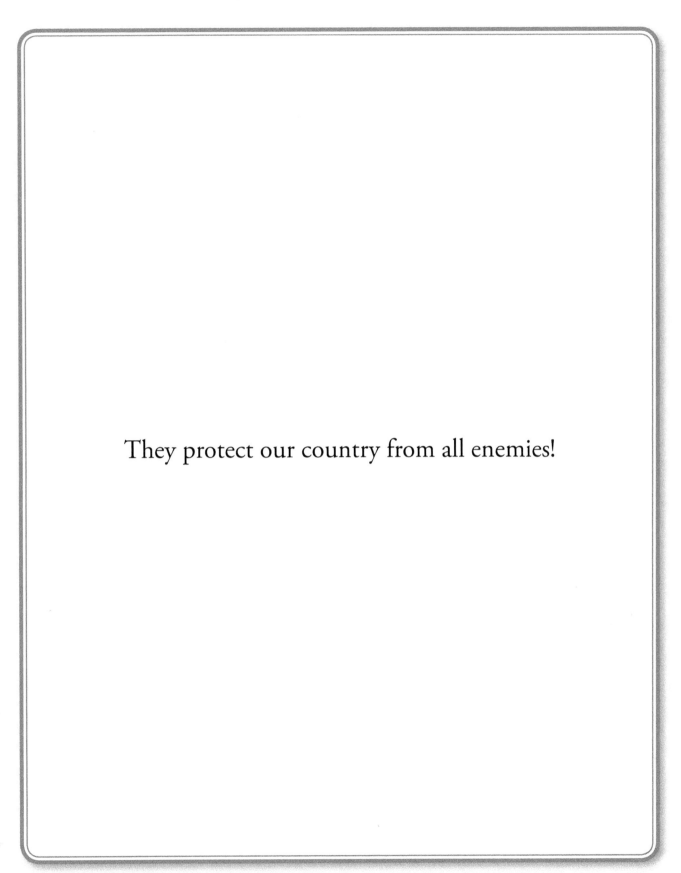

They protect our country from all enemies!

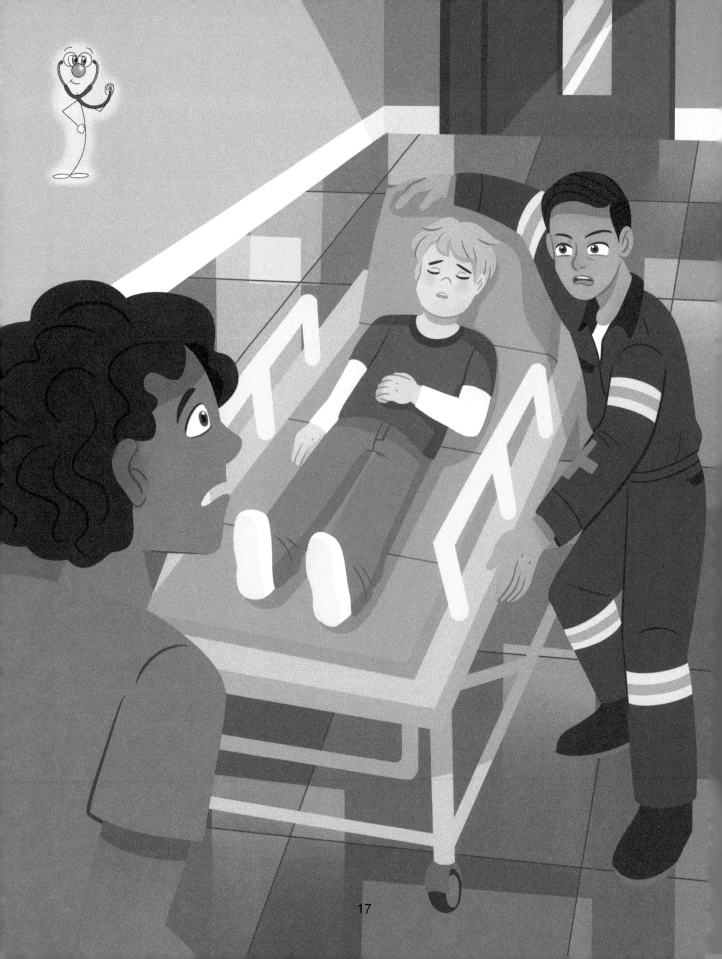

No Head Fred said, "Do this instead. Send thanks to a nurse, doctor, or EMT…"

They will use medicine and care to take away your malady!

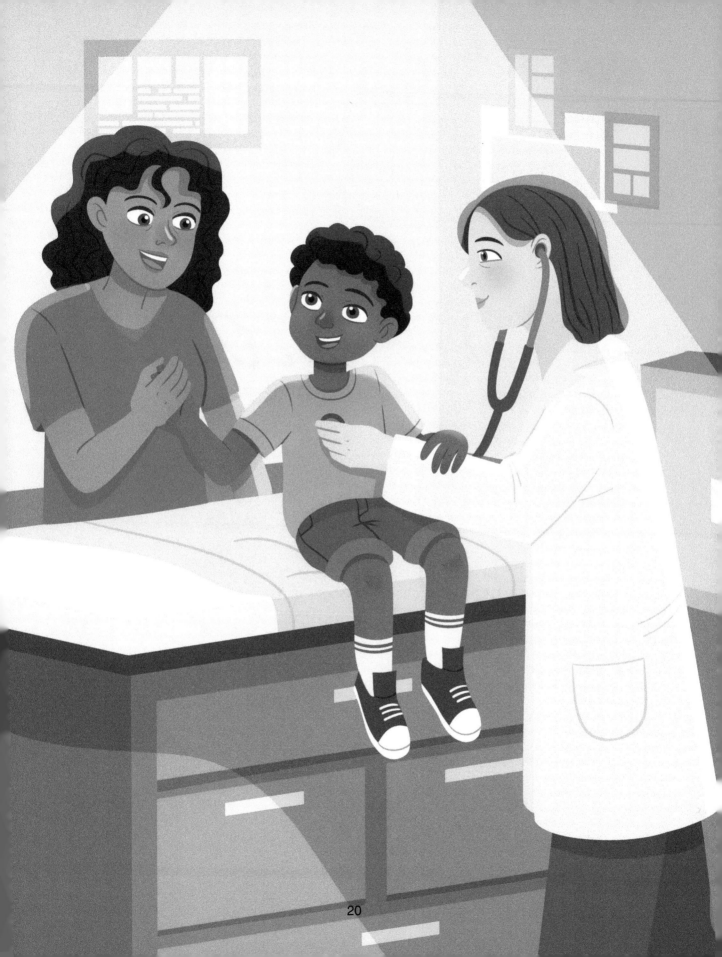

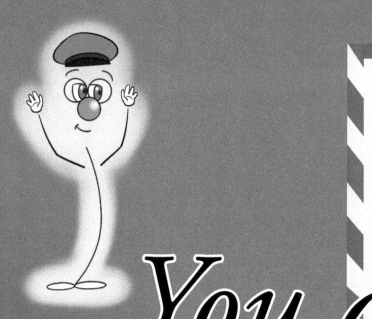

You did it!

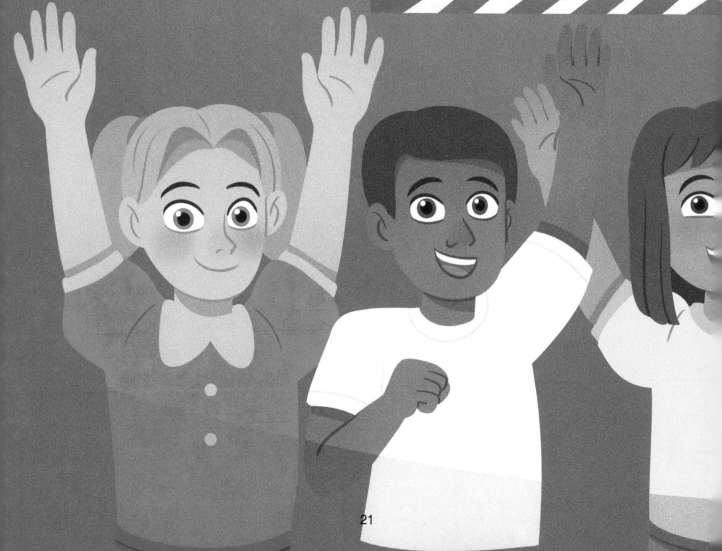

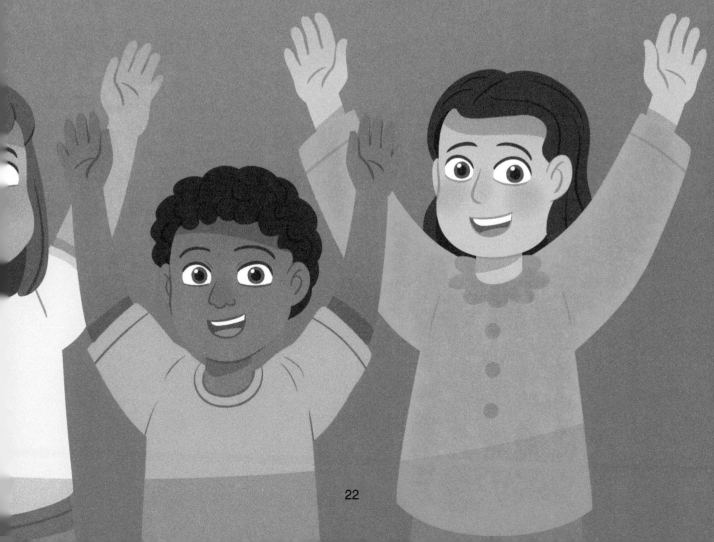

Yay!

About the Author

Stephanie's dream was to write and publish a book. She used her childhood drawing to write children's books to help kids learn. She is a US army veteran. She has a BA in English literature. She has two grown boys. She enjoys reading and sports.

CPSIA information can be obtained
at www.ICGtesting.com
Printed in the USA
LVHW072134151219
640615LV00017B/496/P